ADDYZ

(Sex Pill For Men)

Ultimate guide to maintaining increase sperm count,

enhance libido and increase stamina in bed

Bruce Herbst

1

CHAPTER 1

ADDYZOA

Addyzoa is known to be a sexual medication for male, and it's basically prescribed for those who have issues with poor sexual performances and those whose semen are not sufficient enough. It can as well be liken to an antioxidant based medication responsible for semen production and also helps in enhancing proper function of the male reproductive part.

Likewise, this medication functions to stop the reduction of sperm cell damage.

Various herbs are used in formulating this medication and

as such helps in increasing testosterone level without any complication.

It's also polyherbal in nature; this means that it contains Levo-dopa which is basically responsible for semen parameter improvement in male fertility.

This medication functions for the following use:

Low sperm count

Poor movement of sperm cells

Abnormal or poor sperm morphology

Dosage form of this medication:

This medication is encapsulated; it means it will be seen in a capsule form

Administer a capsule of this medication twice daily for about 3 months (90 days) should your count goes above 10mil/ml.

Administer 2 capsules of this medication twice daily for about 3 months (90 days) should your count goes below 10mil/ml.

USES OF ADDYZOA

This medication is usually prescribed in the following conditions:

Low sperm count

Poor movement of sperm cells

Abnormal or poor sperm morphology

It's a spermatogenic antioxidant

It shrinks the possibility of sperm cell damage

It relieves stress

It promotes sperm cell

It enhances sperm motility

The result shows its effectiveness after its being administered for about 2 weeks, you will get to see your sperm cells rising from the previous figure (this will be deduced from your laboratory result)

MOVEMENT OF SPERM WITH ADDYZOA USE

This medication is indicated for use in treating poor sperm cell motility, after taking your prescribe dose of this medication, it improves semen motility significantly in men with idiopathic OATs after administering this medication for 3 months.

ERECTILE DYSFUNCTION AND SPERM CELL MOTILITY

This medication is as well indicated for the treatment of erectile dysfunction, should you don't have a stable or perfect erection, this medication plays such a vital role in driving sexual libido and as such enhance sexual performances.

This medication can be used only by an adult who has attained the age of 18 years and above.

After administering your dose, you are certain of erection and sperm motility. This medication works perfectly well when you follow the prescribe doses given to you by your health care professional.

Addyzoa is taken by mouth; but you can take this capsule before or after sexual activity.

It can as well be administered 30 minutes to 4 hours before bed.

This medication treats erectile dysfunction and impotency in man, this capsule also successfully helps in maintaining and achieving sexual activities.

This capsule takes about 5 hours for it to work effectively in the body system, this implies that after being sexually arouse, the erection should last no longer than 4 hours

after taken a dose of this medication.

CHAPTER 2

HOW THIS MEDICATION CAN EFECTIVELY

WORK FASTER

To making this medication work faster, it must be taken on an empty stomach to see its positive effect, if consumed with a fat food meal, its action will be delayed and it then becomes less effective as expected.

THE TIME IT TAKES TO WORK IN THE BODY

The drug level decreases with time within few hours, but normally, it takes about 24 hours for this medication to be removed completely from the body system.

CHAPTER 3

SIDE EFFECTS

This medication has little or no side effect, some recorded side effects are:

Slight headache

Dizziness

Nausea

Vomiting

Indigestion

THINGS TO DO TO RELIEVE ADDYZOA SIDE EFFECTS

Often time, the side effect of this medication goes off by itself after taken this capsule. In case you feel dizzy or suffer mild headache, relax a little while, that settles it. Alcohol should not be administered after or before taking this capsule. Turn off any bright light around you, with this headache and light sensitivity will be reduced. Also, you can as well take analgesic to take off pains. If you feel indigestion after taking this pill, ensure you take in little food or snacks. The following will be noticed should this medication is administered at a higher dosage:

Flushing

Indigestion

Nasal congestion

Vision changes

Should higher doses of this medication causes any side effects or leads to any unwanted complication, speak to your health professional to lower your dose as soon as possible.

DOSES OF ADDYZOA

The doses prescribed by your health care professional are based on the following factors:

Age

Kidney or liver issue

Other medical condition

Medication taking

ADDYZOA ERECTILE DYSFUNCTION DOSE

This medication dose (Addyzoa) for Erectile Dysfunction (ED) is a capsule daily. Take it 30 minutes before bed time. You should not use above a capsule of this medication daily for the treatment of ED.

CHAPTER 4

PREMATURE EJACULATION

This can be likening to being a state or an unwanted state where a man comes or ejaculates quickly or sooner than he or his partner wants to. This condition premature ejaculation (PE) takes place infrequently; you've got nothing to be concern with.

Should this condition (premature ejaculation) becomes an issue and ejaculation happens so rapidly or quickly than expected, even before you begin to play on bed (intercourse) or shortly after you begin to play, this is known to be a medical condition called **Premature**

Ejaculation.

The condition has mostly common phenomenon, this imply that in a real sexual issue. It has been researched that about 1 out of 3 men suffers this course (premature ejaculation). This condition (premature ejaculation) happen for various reasons, it could either be:

Psychological

Biological or

Both

Most men do not want to discuss this issue with families or friends, this is because it sounds so embarrassing. But now, be of good cheers, this guide will put you through what is needed as it is a much treatable condition.

To ensure that you can be a better man in bed, between you and your beloved partner, many medications, sexual techniques and even some psychological counseling exists causing a reasonable delay in ejaculation.

For men, this medical condition, premature ejaculation can be solved with treatment combinations.

SYMPTOMS OF PREMATURE EJACULATION

Some signs will quickly been seen if you suffer from this medical condition known as premature ejaculation, the ejaculation takes place before you and your partner wish for the act (sex) to happen, causing stress, concern and embarrassment.

Consequently, this issue occur practically and during coital reflex (sexual interaction), this also includes getting masturbated.

This medical condition (Premature ejaculation) is classified into 2 major categories namely:

Lifelong (primary) premature ejaculation

Acquired (secondary) premature ejaculation

Lifelong (primary) premature ejaculation

You will get to notice the following features:

Always or nearly always, if it occurs within a minute after vaginal penetration

If you are not able to delay ejaculation during vaginal

penetrations

To develop or development of some negative attributes which are sometimes personal such as:

Stress

Frustration

Tendency of avoiding sexual intimacy

Acquired (secondary) premature ejaculation

This occur after which one has had a lovely time (successful and satisfying sexual intercourses) in recent time with no ejaculatory dysfunctions

ADDYZOA USE PRECAUTION

Call or talk to your health care professional before taken this capsule, should you suffer any medical condition, this medication should not be administered, it may affect your health and conditions such as:

Allergic reaction to certain drugs like sildenafil or Viagra

Stroke

Heart issues

Heart problem

Hypertension

Hypotension

Physical abnormalities affecting penis

Blood cell problems

Optic nerve issues

Kidney issues

Retinitis

Liver problem

Kidney problem

Peptic ulcer

Breastfeeding

ABOUT THE AUTHOR

This book author is named **Bruce Herbst** is a great Health care provider and a notable writer of our time, he uses individualized knowledge to put down this basic guide.

ACKNOWLEDGEMENT

Glory to God for this success of this project, kudos to family and friends, you are all the best.

Printed in Great Britain
by Amazon

27750753R00020